Jaypee's Video Atlas of
BEDSIDE CARDIOLOGY

System requirements:

- Operating System – Windows Vista or above
- Recommended Web Browser – Google Chrome and Mozilla Firefox
- Essential plugins – Java and Flash player
  - Facing problems in viewing content – it may be your system does not have java enabled.
  - If Videos do not show up – it may be the system requires Flash player or need to manage flash setting. To learn more about flash setting click on the link in the help section.
  - You can test java and flash by using the links from the help section of the CD/DVD.

Accompanying CD/DVD-ROM is playable only in Computer and not in DVD player.

CD/DVD has Autorun function – it may take few seconds to load on your computer. If it does not works for you then follow the steps below to access the contents manually:

- Click on my computer
- Select the CD/DVD drive and click open/explore – this will show list of files in the CD/DVD
- Find and double click file – "launch.html"

Jaypee's Video Atlas of
BEDSIDE CARDIOLOGY

Atul Luthra MD DNB
Cardio-Diabetologist
Fortis C-DOC
Gurgaon, Haryana, India
dratulluthra@gmail.com
www.atulluthra.in

Foreword
JPS Sawhney

JAYPEE The Health Sciences Publisher
New Delhi | London | Philadelphia | Panama

Jaypee Brothers Medical Publishers (P) Ltd

Headquarters
Jaypee Brothers Medical Publishers (P) Ltd
4838/24, Ansari Road, Daryaganj
New Delhi 110 002, India
Phone: +91-11-43574357
Fax: +91-11-43574314
Email: jaypee@jaypeebrothers.com

Overseas Offices

J.P. Medical Ltd
83, Victoria Street, London
SW1H 0HW (UK)
Phone: +44 20 3170 8910
Fax: +44 (0)20 3008 6180
Email: info@jpmedpub.com

Jaypee Medical Inc.
325 Chestnut Street
Suite 412, Philadelphia, PA 19106, USA
Phone: + 267-519-9789
Email: jpmed.us@gmail.com

Jaypee Brothers Medical Publishers (P) Ltd
Bhotahity, Kathmandu
Nepal
Phone: +977-9741283608
Email: kathmandu@jaypeebrothers.com

Jaypee-Highlights medical publishers Inc
City of Knowledge, Bld. 237, Clayton
Panama City, Panama
Phone: +1 507-301-0496
Fax: +1 507-301-0499
Email: cservice@jphmedical.com

Jaypee Brothers Medical Publishers (P) Ltd
17/1-B Babar Road, Block-B, Shaymali
Mohammadpur, Dhaka-1207
Bangladesh
Mobile: +08801912003485
Email: jaypeedhaka@gmail.com

Website: www.jaypeebrothers.com
Website: www.jaypeedigital.com

Inquiries for bulk sales may be solicited at: jaypee@jaypeebrothers.com

Jaypee's Video Atlas of Bedside Cardiology

First Edition: **2016**

ISBN 978-93-5250-177-9

Printed at Ajanta Offset & Packagings Ltd., New Delhi

Dedicated to

My parents
Ms Prem Lata Luthra
and
Mr Prem Prakash Luthra
who bless me from heaven

FOREWORD

With the widespread availability of sophisticated cutting-edge technology in the field of cardiology, the clinician's approach towards the diagnosis of heart disease has undergone a paradigm shift. These days, patients on arrival to the hospital are sometimes directly wheeled into the noninvasive cardiology department or even into the catheterization laboratory without anyone bothering to place a stethoscope on the precordium of the patient. This is an unhealthy sign since a wealth of vital information is available at the bedside of the patient, which is inadvertently lost.

I must compliment Atul Luthra for this brilliant effort to discuss the clinical examination of the patient and to compile audio clippings of the various heart sounds and murmurs. He has also given a masterly account of the technical aspects of performing electrocardiography and echocardiography. Students preparing for their examinations, resident doctors looking after patients in cardiology wards and paramedical personnel working in noninvasive cardiology units are bound to benefit from this video atlas. I wish Atul and his excellent work all the very best.

JPS Sawhney MD DM
Chairman
Department of Cardiology
Sir Ganga Ram Hospital
New Delhi, India

PREFACE

Three decades ago, I learnt the tips and tricks of clinical cardiology from astute clinicians, at the bedside of patients. Nowadays, cardiology is often taught by means of sophisticated investigative techniques on echocardiography machines, in electrophysiology units as well as inside catheterization laboratories. Nevertheless, a relevant medical history coupled with a meticulous physical examination are indispensible tools, in order to mentally construct a plausible clinical diagnosis of heart disease. Moreover, simple bedside investigations such as electrocardiography (ECG) and echocardiography (ECHO) have withstood the test of time as cost-effective investigation tools in resource-sensitive settings.

It gives me immense pleasure to present to you *Jaypee's Video Atlas of Bedside Cardiology*. The atlas consists of four modules as separate CDs, which cover the different aspects of bedside cardiology. The first module deals with the general examination of the patient and the specific examination of the precordium. The second module deals with the heart sounds and various murmurs, wherein audiovisual technology has been used to appreciate the subtle nuances of cardiac auscultation. The third and fourth modules are devoted to the technique of recording an electrocardiogram (ECG) and performing echocardiography (ECHO), respectively.

Having had the proud privilege of writing four books on cardiology namely *ECG Made Easy, ECHO Made Easy, Tips and Tricks in Bedside Cardiology* and *50 Cases in Clinical Cardiology: A Problem Solving Approach*, I sincerely hope that this video atlas will rekindle the romance between the physician and bedside cardiology. This video atlas should be most useful for students preparing for their examinations, resident doctors looking after patients in cardiology wards and paramedical personnel working in noninvasive cardiology departments.

Atul Luthra

ACKNOWLEDGMENTS

I am extremely grateful to:

- My respected professors, who taught me the science and art of bedside clinical cardiology.
- My esteemed patients, whose clinical examination and investigation results made me wiser.
- My dear students, whose generous appreciation of my books stimulates me to do even more.
- M/s Jaypee Brothers Medical Publishers (P) Ltd, New Delhi, India, for reposing their unflinching faith in me.

CONTENTS

Video **1**

Clinical Examination of the Cardiovascular System

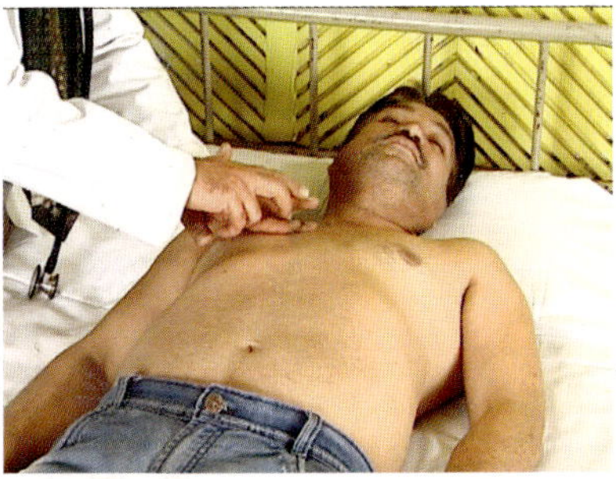

- Auscultation of the heart is not the be all and end all of clinical examination of the cardiovascular system (CVS).
- One should ideally begin with the general physical examination (GPE) of the patient.
- Often the first thing to notice on examination is the built and stature of the patient.
- For instance in children with congenital heart disease, there is growth retardation.
- Rheumatic valvular heart disease in common among women of child-bearing age.
- In overweight individuals coronary artery disease is common, often associated with diabetes, hypertension and dyslipidemia.
- In Marfan syndrome we notice a tall, slender patient with long arms and fingers.
- The general physical examination (GPE) as usual, begins with looking for anemia, cyanosis, jaundice, clubbing and pedal edema.
- Anemia causes tachycardia, bounding pulses and wide pulse pressure, sometimes associated with high-output heart failure.
- Cyanosis is seen with congenital heart disease, and chronic lung disease (corpulmonale).
- A tinge of jaundice is observed due to hepatic congestion in case of right-heart failure.
- Clubbing of fingers is a feature of left-to-right shunt, bacterial endocarditis as well as suppurative lung disease.
- Pitting edema around the ankles is an indicator of congestive heart failure. It is associated with hepatomegaly and engorged neck veins.

- The periorbital region must be examined carefully. In myxedema (hypothyroidism) there is puffiness while in Grave's disease (hyperthyroidism) there is exophthalmos.
- In patients with premature coronary artery disease, there may be xanthelasma on the eyelids due to hyperlipidemia or arcus senilis around the cornea.
- The neck is examined for jugular venous pressure (JVP), the thyroid gland, position of the trachea and signs of insulin resistance.
- A raised jugular venous pressure (JVP) with normal waves indicates fluid overload or right heart failure.
- A raised JVP with absent waves indicates superior vena cava (SVC) obstruction.
- A raised JVP that rises further on inspiration (Kussmaul's sign) is observed in case of constrictive pericarditis or restrictive cardiomyopathy.
- The "a" wave is tall in pulmonary valve disease, absent in atrial fibrillation, while cannon "a" waves are seen in atrioventricular dissociation.
- The "y" descent is rapid in tricuspid regurgitation, absent in cardiac tamponade and deep in case of constrictive pericarditis.
- The thyroid gland is enlarged in Grave's disease (hyperthyroidism). There may be a fine tremor, tachycardia, exophthalmos and an audible bruit over the gland.
- The trachea may be displaced to either side with shift of the mediastinum. It is pulled to the same side by pulmonary collapse or pushed to the other side by pleural effusion.
- Signs of insulin resistance around the neck are purplish velvety areas in the skin folds (acanthosis nigricans) and skin tags (acrochordon).
- The pulse is examined for rate, rhythm, volume and character; the radial pulse for rate and rhythm, the brachial pulse for volume and character.
- A low-volume pulse (pulsus parvus) is observed in aortic stenosis and in any low-output state such as congestive heart failure or cardiac tamponade.
- A high-volume pulse (collapsing pulse) is observed in aortic regurgitation and in any high-output state such as anemia, thyrotoxicosis or arteriovenous fistula.
- A pulse with a double-peak (pulsus bisferiens) is a feature of combined aortic stenosis and regurgitation, and of hypertrophic cardiomyopathy.
- A pulse that falls in volume on inspiration (pulsus paradoxus) is observed in case of constrictive pericarditis and cardiac tamponade.
- The peripheral pulses are examined for an audible bruit over the carotid arteries and diminished pulsations over the dorsalis pedis arteries.
- Examination of the precordium begins with inspection. The precordium is inspected for surgical scars, skeletal deformities and visible pulsations.

- A scar of sternotomy in a child points towards an operated congenital heart disease, while that in an adult indicates prior coronary artery bypass graft (CABG) surgery.
- Common skeletal deformities are pectus excavatum of the sternum and kyphoscoliosis of the spine. These deformities can potentially displace the apex beat.
- Pulsations in the suprasternal notch and the epigastrium are visible in aneurysmal dilatation of the ascending and descending aorta respectively.
- The first and foremost reason for palpation of the precordium is to locate the apex beat and to assess its character.
- The apex beat is the lowermost and outermost point of the cardiac pulsation. It is normally located in the 5th intercostal space in the midclavicular line.
- The apex beat is difficult to locate if there is any intervening tissue between the palpating finger and the cardiac impulse.
- Examples of intervening tissue are fat in obesity, muscle in athletic built, air in pulmonary emphysema and fluid in pericardial effusion.
- The apex beat is displaced downwards and outwards in case of left ventricular dilatation. It is displaced to the left by pectus excavatum and kyphoscoliosis.
- Pulmonary disease can also displace the apex beat. Lung collapse pulls the apex beat to the same side while pleural effusion pushes the apex beat to the opposite side.
- Accordingly, reasons for a right-sided apex beat are mirror-image dextrocardia, a left-sided pleural effusion or a right-sided lung collapse.
- The apex beat may be localized or diffuse and tapping or heaving in character. It is localized in left ventricular hypertrophy and diffuse in ventricular enlargement.
- The apex beat is tapping in mitral stenosis and heaving in mitral regurgitation. The heave is sustained in aortic stenosis and ill-sustained in case of mitral regurgitation.
- The next reason for cardiac palpation is to feel a parasternal heave in case of right ventricular hypertrophy, by placing the edge of the palm to the left of the sternum.
- A cardiac murmur greater than grade 4/6 in intensity, is palpated as a thrill. The thrill of aortic stenosis and mitral regurgitation radiate towards the neck and axilla respectively.
- Percussion of the precordium has specific indications. The area of cardiac dullness is enlarged in case of pericardial effusion.
- In case of left ventricular failure, an area of dullness is percussed over the right lung base, due to the presence of a pleural effusion.
- When the lower edge of the liver is palpable, careful percussion of the upper edge can differentiate between an enlarged liver from a liver that's pushed down by emphysema.

Video 2

Auscultation of the Heart for Sounds and Murmurs

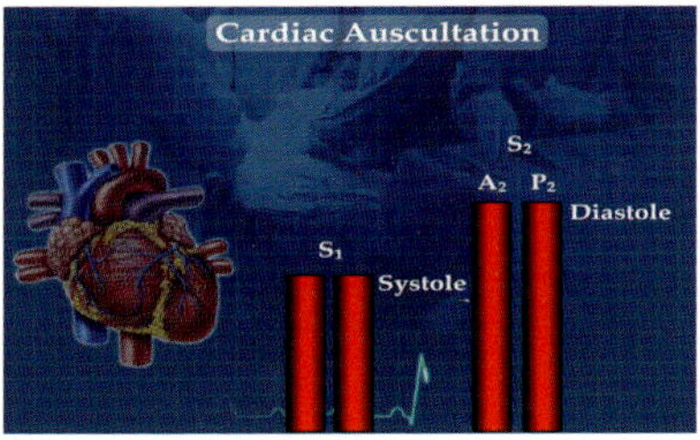

- The art and skill of cardiac auscultation, has been traditionally passed down from expert teachers in medical colleges to gullible students.
- However, competence in this field of expertise remains extremely variable, largely because it cannot be quantified by objective parameters.
- In this module of learning, digital audiovisual technology has been used which will enable the amateur cardiologist to appreciate subtle nuances of auscultation.
- Auscultation of the heart begins with appreciation of the two normal heart sounds namely first heart sound (S1) and second heart sound (S2).
- Together, the S1 and S2 produce a rhythm that sounds like "lub-dub lub-dub lub-dub".
- The S1 is produced by closure of the mitral valve followed by the tricuspid valve, at the onset of ventricular systole.
- The intensity of S1 depends upon the distance between the mitral leaflets at the onset of systole, which in turn, depends on the diastolic filling time.
- When the diastolic filling time is short, the distance between the mitral leaflets is long and they snap together loudly.
- Causes of a loud S1 are mitral stenosis, tachycardia and a short PR interval.
- When the diastolic filling time is long, the distance between the mitral leaflets is short and they snap together softly.
- Causes of a soft S1 are mitral regurgitation, bradycardia and a long PR interval.
- The mitral and tricuspid components of S1 are usually inseparable. Splitting of S1 occurs when the tricuspid component is delayed.

- Causes of a split S1 are right bundle branch block and Ebstein anomaly.
- The intensity of S1 is variable if the diastolic period varies from beat-to-beat.
- Causes of a variable S1 are atrial fibrillation and atrioventricular dissociation.
- The S2 is normally split and produced by closure of the aortic valve followed by the pulmonary valve, at the end of ventricular systole.
- The intensity of the aortic component (A2) and pulmonary component (P2) of S2 depends upon the rate of deceleration of retrograde flow.
- The A2 is loud in systemic hypertension and in aneurysmal dilatation of the aorta, while it is soft in calcific aortic stenosis and absent in aortic atresia.
- The P2 is loud in pulmonary hypertension and in dilatation of the pulmonary artery, while it is soft in pulmonary stenosis and absent in pulmonary atresia.
- The S2 is normally split with closure of the aortic valve being followed by the closure of the pulmonary valve, at the end of ventricular systole.
- The splitting of S2 is better appreciated during inspiration because increase in venous return delays the pulmonary component or P2.
- Wide splitting of S2 is observed in right bundle branch block (delayed right ventricular activation), pulmonary stenosis (prolonged right ventricular ejection) and in mitral regurgitation (short left ventricular ejection time).
- Reverse or paradoxical splitting of S2 is where A2 follows P2. In that case, the splitting narrows down in inspiration when P2 is delayed.
- Reverse splitting of S2 is observed in left bundle branch block (delayed left ventricular activation), aortic stenosis (prolonged left ventricular ejection) and in aortic valve regurgitation (long left ventricular ejection time).
- Pacing of the right ventricle by an external pacemaker or pre-excitation by an accessory bypass tract also cause reverse splitting of S2.
- Wide and fixed splitting of S2 that does not widen further during inspiration occurs in atrial septal defect. The shunt abolishes the effect of respiration on atrial filling.
- Fixed splitting of S2 also occurs in right ventricular dysfunction. This is because inspiration cannot augment ventricular filling any further.
- The third heart sound (S3) is a soft sound that follows S2. It is produced by a sudden halt in diastolic ventricular filling and coincides with the "y" descent of the jugular pulsation.
- Physiological S3 is heard in high-output states, valvular regurgitation and cardiac shunt. Pathological S3 is heard in left ventricular systolic dysfunction.

- The pericardial knock (PK) resembles S3 but it occurs earlier and is sharper in character. It is heard in case of constrictive pericarditis.
- The fourth heart sound (S4) is a high-pitched sound that precedes S1. It is produced by atrial contraction and coincides with the "a" wave of the jugular venous pulse.
- The S4 is always pathological and indicates impaired left ventricular relaxation as in case of systemic hypertension, aortic stenosis and restrictive/hypertrophic cardiomyopathy.
- The opening snap (OS) is produced by sudden tensing of the anterior mitral leaflet at the end of isovolumic relaxation and beginning of ventricular filling.
- It is typically audible in mitral stenosis and indicates pliability of the valve. The opening snap is absent in calcific stenosis and after mitral valvotomy.
- A short interval between the S2 and OS indicates high left atrial pressure and severe mitral stenosis, since ventricular filling begins early after S2.
- The tumor plop (TP) of left atrial myxoma resembles the OS of mitral stenosis. It is produced by prolapse of the myxoma into the mitral valve orifice.
- An ejection click (EC) is a sharp sound that precedes the ejection systolic murmur of aortic or pulmonary valvular stenosis.
- It is produced by sudden halt of maximal excursion of the valve leaflets and indicates end of isovolumic contraction with onset of ejection.
- Presence of ejection click indicates pliability of the valve, differentiates valvular from infundibular stenosis and rules out innocent flow murmurs.
- In case of mitral valve prolapse, single or multiple nonejection click(s) are audible in mid-systole, indicating sudden tensing of the redundant anterior mitral leaflet.
- A pansystolic murmur begins with S1, spans the entire systole and ends with S2. Causes of pansystolic murmur are mitral/ tricuspid regurgitation and ventricular septal defect.
- In mitral regurgitation (MR), the murmur stops short of S2 and is only early systolic if the MR is acute or severe, since high left atrial pressure impedes flow in late systole.
- Similarly in ventricular septal defect (VSD), the murmur is only early systolic if the VSD is large in size, muscular in location or associated with pulmonary arterial hypertension.
- An ejection mid-systolic murmur is diamond-shaped and peaks in mid-systole. Causes of an ejection murmur are aortic and pulmonary valve stenosis.
- In aortic stenosis (AS), the mid-systolic murmur may be preceded by an ejection click, accompanied by a palpable thrill and it radiates towards the neck.
- A late-systolic murmur is heard in case of mitral valve prolapse, due to late-systolic mitral regurgitation. It is preceded by a single or multiple nonejection click(s).

- An early-diastolic murmur just follows the S2 and stops short of S1. Causes of an early-diastolic murmur are aortic and pulmonary valve regurgitation.
- The early-diastolic murmur of aortic regurgitation (AR) is decrescendo in nature and it is high-pitched, soft and blowing in character.
- The murmur of AR is best heard over the parasternal area with the diaphragm of the stethoscope firmly pressed and the patient sitting up leaning forward.
- The early-diastolic murmur of pulmonary regurgitation (PR) with a loud P2 indicates pulmonary arterial hypertension. It is known as the Grahm-Steel murmur.
- A mid-diastolic murmur follows the opening snap and undergoes accentuation before S1. Causes of a mid-diastolic murmur are mitral and tricuspid stenosis.
- The length of the mid-diastolic murmur correlates with the severity of mitral stenosis (MS). Presystolic accentuation is absent in the presence of atrial fibrillation.
- The mid-diastolic murmur of mitral stenosis is harsh and low-pitched, rough and rumbling in character.
- The murmur of MS is best heard over the mitral area with the bell of the stethoscope lightly placed and the patient lying in the left-lateral position.
- A late-diastolic murmur occurs in case of left atrial myxoma and follows the tumor plop. The murmur changes in character with the position of the patient.
- Besides mitral stenosis and atrial myxoma, other causes of a mid or late diastolic murmur are mitral leaflet fluttering in case of aortic regurgitation (Austin Flint murmur) and increased diastolic flow (mitral regurgitation and ventricular septal defect).
- A continuous murmur occurs throughout systole, crosses the S2 and spills over into diastole. It has the same character in systole and diastole.
- Causes of a continuous murmur are patent ductus arteriosus (PDA), aortopulmonary window (APW), ruptured aneurysm sinus of Valsalva (SOV), arteriovenous fistula (AVF), coarctation of aorta, venous hum and mammary soufflé.
- The continuous murmur of PDA is maximum around the S2. It is known as machinery murmur or the Gibson's murmur. When pulmonary hypertension develops, the murmur remains only systolic.
- A systolo-diastolic murmur is a combination of a systolic murmur and diastolic murmur. It has a different character in systole and diastole.
- Causes of a systolo-diastolic murmur are aortic stenosis with regurgitation (rheumatic heart disease), ventricular septal defect with aortic regurgitation (supracristal VSD) and atrial septal defect with mitral stenosis (Lutembacher syndrome).

- Other sounds that may be heard over the precordium are pericardial rub (pericarditis), mediastinal crunch (mediastinal emphysema), Means-Lerman scratch (thyrotoxicosis).
- The intensity and character of a murmur may change with the position of the patient, the phase of respiration and performance of certain maneuvers.
- Murmurs that may change with the position of the patient are those of mitral valve prolapse, atrial myxoma and bacterial endocarditis.
- During inspiration, increase in venous return to the right atrium increases the intensity of murmurs arising from the right side of the heart and decreases the intensity of left-sided murmurs. The reverse happens during expiration.
- An exception to this rule is the ejection click of pulmonary valve stenosis that reduces in intensity during the phase of inspiration.
- Maneuvers that reduce the size of the left ventricular cavity, reduce the intensity of most left-sided murmurs. These maneuvers are standing, Valsalva and nitroglycerine.
- Conversely, maneuvers that increase the size of the left ventricular cavity, increase the intensity of most left-sided murmurs. These are squatting, hand-grip and propranolol.
- Exceptions to this rule are the murmurs of mitral valve prolapse (MVP) and hypertrophic obstructive cardiomyopathy (HOCM) that are left-sided murmurs but become louder and longer with maneuvers that reduce the size of the left ventricular cavity.
- This is because reduction in the size of the left ventricular cavity, increases the degree of mitral leaflet buckling and outflow tract obstruction respectively.

Video **3**

The Technique of Recording an Electrocardiogram

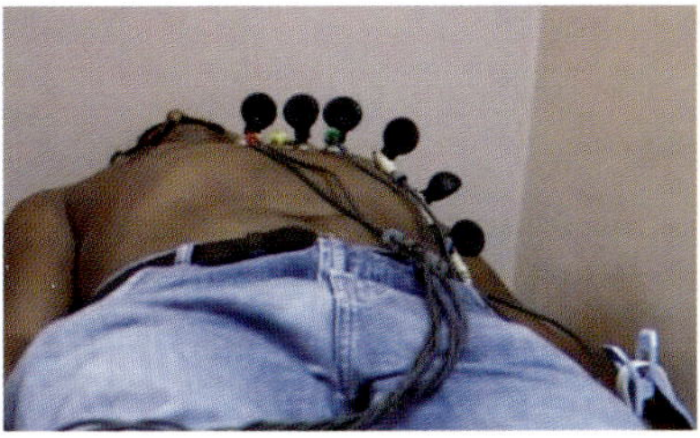

- We are living in an era wherein there have been several technological advancements in the field of diagnostic cardiology.
- However, the electrocardiogram (ECG) has withstood the test of time as a dependable investigation for the initial evaluation of a patient with suspected or established heart disease.
- Moreover, it is a simple, useful, cost-effective and readily available diagnostic modality, even is centers that lack advanced diagnostic facilities.
- All that recording of an ECG requires is a comfortable couch on which the patient can lie down and a good-quality ECG machine.
- In order to obtain a good ECG recording, the first and foremost requisite is proper preparation of the patient.
- The patient is made to lie down on a couch of sufficient size. The wrists, ankles and the precordium are exposed for application of electrodes.
- The room temperature must be comfortable for the patient and there should be no external electrical circuits besides the ECG machine.
- The patient must be calm and relaxed, while the respiration should be slow and shallow. This prevents drifting of the baseline while recording
- For recording, electrodes are placed on the wrists, the ankles and on standard positions over the precordium.
- The patient cable consists of 10 leads; each lead carries an electrode on its tip.
- In all there are 10 electrodes; 4 are placed on the limbs and 6 electrodes are placed over the precordial area.
- The limb electrodes are secured in position by clamps. Each clamp has a flat metallic plate for contact and a groove into which the electrode fits.

- The chest electrodes are secured in position by rubber-bulbs. Each bulb has a cup-shaped metallic piece and a groove into which the electrode fits.
- Before securing the electrode to its position, the skin is smeared with jelly to maintain good skin contact and to prevent vibration artefacts.
- The limb electrodes are color-coded as follows: Black right leg (RL); green left leg (LL); red right arm (RA); yellow left arm (LA).
- The chest electrodes are marked V1 to V6 and placed as follows: V1-to the right of sternum; V2-to the left of sternum; V3-between V2 and V4; V4-midclavicular line; V5-anterior axillary line; V6-mid-axillary line (V4 to V6 5th intercostal space).
- The 10 leads of the patient cable converge on a junction box, from where a single lead emerges that fits into the socket on the ECG machine.
- Normally, the ECG deflection is standardized to 10 mm and the recording is done at a paper speed of 25 mm/sec. Vibrations are automatically filtered.
- However, during ECG recording, certain technical artefacts and trouble-shooters are inadvertently encountered.
- Vibration artifact can occur because of interference from electrical mains or due to lack of proper insulation by jelly.
- Recording the graph at a speed of 50 mm/sec can be mistaken for bradycardia. Overdamping can cause low voltages while underdamping leads to overshoot.
- Baseline drifting is caused by loose contact between the electrode and the skin while gross baseline wandering is due to deep breathing by the patient.

Video **4**

The Technique of Performing an Echocardiogram

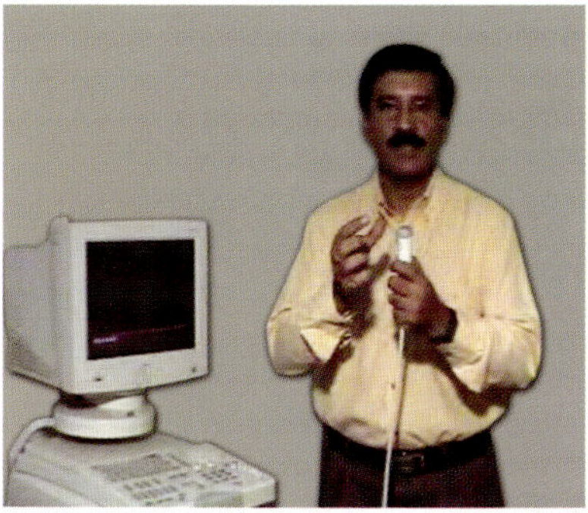

- In recent years, the application of ultrasound has increased exponentially, in several fields of clinical medicine.
- In fact, ultrasonography is today accepted as the fifth dimension of clinical examination after inspection, palpation, percussion and auscultation.
- Echocardiography is the application of ultrasound to examine the heart. It is a practical, noninvasive, cost-effective and reliable investigative tool.
- More and more physicians are these days performing or requesting for an echo to diagnose or exclude cardiac disease.
- An echo is performed for the diagnosis and assessment of virtually all forms of heart disease including congenital defects, valvular diseases, coronary heart disease, myocardial problems and pericardial disorders.
- Echo provides substantial amount of anatomical and physiological information.
- While still-frames or frozen images provide structural details, dynamic or real-time images convey functional abnormalities.
- Hemodynamic parameters that can be measured by echo are stroke volume, cardiac output, ejection fraction and pulmonary artery pressure.
- The modalities of echo used are two-dimensional (2-D), motion-mode (M-mode) and Doppler echo. Doppler echo includes pulsed-wave (PW), continuous-wave (CW) and color-flow map (CFM).

- All modalities follow the same principle of ultrasound but differ in terms of the manner in which the reflected signal is analyzed and displayed. They are not mutually exclusive but complement each other.
- Echocardiography is generally performed from the transthoracic route (TTE). If this is technically difficult due to the presence of obesity, emphysema or chest deformity, transesophageal echo (TEE) is performed.
- For transthoracic echo (TTE), specific areas on the chest are used, which are known as the standard echo windows.
- Standard echo windows are left parasternal, apical, subcostal and suprasternal. At these areas, there is minimum interference from ribs and lungs.
- Standard echo windows allow comparison between serial echoes performed in the same patient on different occasions.
- For echocardiography, the patient is asked to lie on his left side with the right arm placed along the body and the left arm tucked under the head.
- The transducer houses several piezoelectric crystals that transmit ultrasound waves, which are reflected back and analyzed.
- The transducer (probe) is smeared with insulating jelly and placed on the chest. It has a mark or dot that orients the probe.
- The probe is angulated anteriorly or posteriorly to bring the area of interest into focus and rotated clockwise or counter-clockwise to fine-tune the image.
- Images acquired from different echo windows are used to mentally construct the structure of the heart and to prepare a comprehensive report.
- During echocardiography, transducers having different frequencies are used. One has to strike a balance between resolution and penetration.
- Low frequency probes (3.5 MHz) provide good penetration but low resolution. They are used to evaluate deep structures and in adult subjects.
- High frequency probes (7.5 MHz) provide low penetration but good resolution. They are used to evaluate superficial structures and in children.
- The intensity of reflected ultrasound depends upon the tissue that reflects it. Bone is white, myocardium is gray and air or blood appears black.
- On the display screen, the image appears in the shape of a triangle. The probe is at the apex of the triangle from which multiple lines emerge.
- Accordingly, superficial structures appear on the upper portion of the screen while deep structures appear on the lower portion of the screen.